I0441674

HOW TO LOSE BELLY FAT

Meal plans for ultimate weight loss for men and women in 8 weeks

STEP-BY-STEP GUIDE FOR BURNING BODY FAT

EDWARD CRUZ

Get the free video training course on 30-Day Abs Workout:

https://goo.gl/X70yqF

WHY I WROTE THIS BOOK

Become a better person! It is a call, which people daily address others, but rarely themselves. We urge our subordinates at work that they need to perform their tasks in a more scrupulous way. We encourage our children at home to be wise, instilling the need to overcome complexities of the educational process and other burdens of life. We meddle in a dialogue with friends, proving that if we were them, we would act in a different way though not feeling the real pressure of their situation. However, we actually forget that we need the call for being a better person no less than others do. The inner advice, persistence and personal responsibility for our own future and present are the things we should lay the emphasis on.

I have long been actively promoting a healthy lifestyle. I am a fitness trainer for celebrities, a fitness model, an actor and a businessman. I and my childhood friend, who is also a fitness trainer and a model, have decided to combine our knowledge, summarizing it in this book to improve the life of our readers. You may ask: why do you need this? The answer is trivial - to improve our own lives. But how can you improve your quality of life via improving the lives of absolutely unknown people? - you may ask in turn. Again, the answer is simple - we live in a vast social environment called the planet Earth. A maple leaf falling on one hemisphere bursts the storm on the other hemisphere. In the same way, the actions of one person sets in motion the mechanism of creation or destruction of all human beings on the planet, especially his/her relatives and friends.

We improve our own lives by making your life better, even if it is not fated to meet in person. The reviews of our positive actions wave back to the initiator in order to compensate for the given a hundred times. This motivation has long been available for every wise person, so we have decided to create the informational product of the direct benefit for a reader by combining our efforts. This book provides the structured and accessible description of the mysteries and postulates of building a strong healthy body. After all, a body is largely the basis for clearing any bars, disclosing the inner capacity and achieving what once seemed impossible.

We present the most efficient information, having analyzed the frequently asked questions of our clients, the problems encountered by the seekers of a strong, toned torso and the strength of our experience. In addition, we have assessed a bulk of third-party works, practices, and the tips of popular world sports bloggers. So, we have come to the conclusion that there are two basic types of presenting information such as:

1. The theory intertwined with author's fantasy, which just partially radiates efficient pieces of advice and often conventional, ineffective or even harmful stereotypes.

2. Cold hard facts, which are rather viable in terms of efficiency, detailed and structured, but lacking a clear rationale providing the cause-and-effect relations that explain everything that happens to a person during their fulfillment of the prescribed rules.

We have decided to follow another path and made an exact step-by-step list of actions and minute-by-minute plan per day, together with a reasonable explanation of the processes that occur within the human body during its forming-up and development. The awareness and explanation of what people do, why they do that and how their bodies should respond to their actions, gives the trainees confidence in the safety of the chosen path and better control over the situation. This approach is the most efficient and right one. Being aware of the developments in a particular point of the path, a person will be ready to overcome difficulties with a stronger confidence.

The will of people who just embark on the healthy lifestyle often weakens when stumbling upon the wall of physical fatigue, nervous anger and lack of quick results. However, our scheme, where the invested efforts equal the results, allows you to completely get rid of the chance of failure at each stage and in different situations. Each subsequent step will be spelled out, and the book lines will support you in times of shortage and unaccustomed efforts as the hand of a personal trainer. Absolutely all information is tested personally by us and takes into account the characteristics of people of different stature and sex. Every word and every tip in this book have been tested first-hand and confirmed by people with different metabolic features and age.

The main emphasis will be put on getting rid of excess fat and restoring normal circulation of the natural life support systems. You should not forget about the problems, provoked with an increase in the level of fat in a body. Such problems include type 1 and 2 diabetes, the progression of cardiovascular diseases, complications of the thyroid body operation and many other challenges, depriving you of joys of life and normal human being. All of this is much closer and more real than you think. There is simply no logical explanation of why you should wish yourself something like that. Difficult working conditions, unhealthy heredity traits, losing courage because of stressful situations are just trivial matters, having no control over you and not preventing you from changing yourself right now.

People are the most adaptive creatures on this planet. No other living creature is capable of such a prompt adaptation to changing conditions, the environment or their own progress. Right now you tear off the veil of your uncertainty, distance all the problems associated with the drawbacks in your appearance and become one step closer to a higher level of social perception. The people around you see bright potential in a beautiful, slender, fit person making them treat you with respect and kindness. Despite the fact that an increase in people's recognition leads to improvement of your life, the main factor of the development will be a rise in your own estimation.

Why You Should Read This Book

First and foremost, the book gives you exact step-by-step guide for burning body fat. It is the body fat index not muscle mass or endocrine cells will be burnt if you follow the rules set forth in the book. Besides, you will not lack vitamins, proteins, and carbohydrates. Only pure fat burdening your hips and hideous stomach skin folds will leave you day by day, releasing the true beauty of the muscle mass. Even if your lifestyle has not contributed to the development and formation of dense muscle tissue, the natural muscular frame will look at times better than a fat "life ring."

At the same time, the book gives you a knowledge base about the energy consumption of the body, depending on human activity, peculiarities of metabolism and sex. The book reasons the aspects of the response to changes in daily bad habits, response to change in daily calorie intake, in the regime of heavy undertake or overtake. We will inform you about the importance of taking into account the energy expenses for achieving a certain task. We will specify features of perception of different types of food by a body and its response to the effectiveness of the chosen method of weight loss.

Chapter "Types and Peculiarities of Diets" lists the most popular types of diets, safe application of various methods to lose weight, recommendations for approaches to them and warnings for different categories of trainees. Other tips include the list of ingredients and the peculiarities of their intake, the possible result of certain diets, possible dangers, and pieces of advice to understand whether your body has a positive response to the chosen program. You will also get acquainted with the main errors while being on a diet and reasons for the absence of result for those who like to read through the lines. We will explain how to calculate the personal proportions, ounces, and calories. Besides, you will understand why some people end the diet with success while others daily deprive themselves of something and harm their health in the end.

Chapter "Food for Result" writes out every calorie of the daily meal plan for men with varying degrees of daily load, as well as products which are easily perceived by women and lead to weight loss without weakening the immune system and producing the effect of "rollback", i.e. the return of lost weight immediately after termination of the diet. Several alternative types of diet will be provided taking into account the tastes of different groups of readers. We will prompt how to adjust your daily diet without exhausting the internal organs, but steadily losing weight on schedule. We will add specific harmless and available sports supplements to the list of products.

We will touch upon the issue of targeted load in the context of weight loss and achievement of a thin waist. We will analyze the effect of muscle growth, the general processes of anabolism and why the catabolism is more important for the weight loss. You will find out how and when you should do a cardio workout, power exercises and reveal more details about the aerobic exercises. The information will be secured with conclusions to consolidate the theory and to easily perceive specific tips on losing weight. If you adhere to our description of the basic dogma, you will definitely be successful in having a beautiful and healthy body, worthy of the attention of people who are an example for hundreds of thousands of their followers.

TABLE OF CONTENTS

Why I Wrote This Book

Why You Should Read This Book

Table of Contents

Chapter 1. Body Energy

Chapter 2. Types and Peculiarities of Diets

Chapter 3. Food for Result

Chapter 4. Movement is Life

Chapter 5. Minimum Fat, Maximum Meat

About The Author

CHAPTER 1. BODY ENERGY

Only the most imprudent and irresponsible people do not think about how their body looks. However, not everybody ponders why it looks so. The problem of excess weight, born and spread in recent decades, has not been caused by the collapse of health care. The fact is that sufficiency is transformed into a surplus in the absence of self-control. Hence, the majority of people have no effective methods of self-restraint, and the opportunity for consuming a large amount of calories leads to obesity. We see a detrimental effect, not of the progress, the disadvantages of the health care system or something else, but namely that of the lack of awareness and being able to distinguish between the norm and the overtake. Thus, we are creating a fertile ground for diabetes, coronary heart disease, rheumatic fever and even banal shortness of breath. Energy is, in fact, the process of converting one type of matter to another. In our case, we speak of using the matter (food) in the construction of new cells in our body.

ENERGY IS AN INTEGRAL PART OF LIFE

Human life is simply impossible without the processes of energy metabolism. It does not matter whether you are sitting, standing, boxing or programming an artificial intelligence – all these activities take away some of your energy. The curious thing is that taking into account the individual organs, muscles, or any other part of a body, the brain remains the main energy consumer. Hard to believe, the brain of even the most massive representatives of our species consumes 22-28% of the energy needed for a body per day. The rest "screws" our body by consuming less energy, though they also work 24 hours a day without stopping. Every breath, every beat of the heart, the daily regeneration process, the growth of new cells in the epidermis - all of this requires energy.

Almost all the processes occurring in a body work at a subconscious or cellular level. That is, you do not think about the need to grow a fingernail or to take tears from somewhere when crying. Our body assumes responsibility for all these things using hundreds of thousands of years of evolution experience. A body itself determines what is good or bad, how to redistribute its resources to maintain normal operations. If a body needs fat in order to guarantee its own future security, it will put off this fat. A body does not care how you look, or how you want to look, it is selfish and self-sufficient in terms of its control.

A body is able to perform its own tasks at the expense of energy: to maintain the temperature, to cure wounds or to reproduce. Therefore, it knows what food products contain a maximum amount of the energy and where it can get the needed fuel from. Such fuel can be easily taken from chocolate bars, juicy grilled steaks, sweet donuts or any type of high caloric food. A body is wild about such food products due to their high-calorie content and is ready to eat them as a reserve. Accordingly, the actions that reduce the stocks of calories are perceived by a body as an attack on its property. A body feels great when lying in front of the TV screen, but not when running on a treadmill at 5 am, having a headache. That is why a body emits a specific group of hormones making us think about sex, food, or fatigue to save energy when dealing with these tasks, rather than deliberately losing weight or writing a thesis or addressing the issues of high complexity.

It is easier for our body to solve primitive problems by using a minimum of precious resources. Such a manifestation of laziness is quite negatively perceived in society but is absolutely understandable in terms of the defense mechanisms of a body. Even if you realize that you have enough fat deposits to survive the winter, a body will minimize its consumption, resorting to different tricks. Such audacity leads to the fact that it is very difficult to maintain a slim figure and it is difficult to get rid of excess weight. A body will not easily give up such a valuable resource as fat.

FAT EQUALS ENERGY.

The only right decision you may make in order to lose weight is to consume fewer energy sources your body needs to start to form its reserves. Let us focus on this for a complete understanding of what was said. To lose weight, you need to consume less food (and, therefore, less energy) than your body spends throughout the day. All other versions, including the advertising about miraculous weight-loss schemes, are idle talks not worth your time. Any complicated secret ingredients for diet or methods of dumbbells grip have no special significance. Only the difference between the consumed and spent energy per day (in kcal) is the grain in the field of sports practices, which leads to a reduction in body fat.

Everything is as easy as ABC and does not require a doctor's degree to understand the usual formula of daily energy consumption.

- If you consume **MORE** energy than your body needs for normal operation, the body fat rises.
- If you consume **LESS** energy than your body needs, you lose the fat deposits.

That is, there is no need to add some three components or features of a certain person's metabolism. The whole point is this simple scheme consisting of intake and expenditure. The formula of nutrition with limited energy consumption (kcal) is called a **DIET**. The expenditure may have a passive and an active component.

- The basic expenditure implies energy costs for the processes of a body that you do not control or control partially (breathing, heartbeat, regeneration, natural growth).
- The active expenditure supposes other actions, which are deliberately triggered by conscious human incentive, consciousness (walking, reading, drawing, turning a head, moving a hand, facial expressions, etc.).

BASIC ENERGY EXPENDITURE

The principle of energy costs at the passive expenditure may be perfectly explained through the example of a person in a coma. The passive energy expenditure occurs even without moving, without making any emotional or mental activity. Of course, this expenditure is several times less than when walking, reading or taking other action, but it still happens. This passive expenditure occurs every second throughout your life. The amount of the burned calories will depend on the characteristics of your body. Many factors influence these indicators: age, genetic features, rate of metabolism, sex, etc.

One more interesting conclusion can be made when looking at the muscular athletes. Their muscle mass gives additional power and speed but requires a large energy return instead. If we compare two almost identical persons of the same sex, age, weight, roughly similar rate of metabolism, but one has more muscles while the other has more fat cells, the muscular man will consume more energy. The muscle mass in this context will play into the hands of its owner, giving an advantage in the possible amount of the consumed calories. That is, a person with the muscular athletic body can eat more harmful high-calorie food with a lesser risk to gain fat deposits. Accordingly, a huge muscular guy who is heavier than the previous athlete can eat even more high-calorie food.

Conclusion: The more muscles your body has, the more energy it consumes and the simpler it is to keep yourself fit.

However, the actions taking place outside of our consciousness still can be influenced. Although the internal processes are being regulated without our direct order, it is possible to stimulate the hormonal processes by two commonly used methods:

1. The first method is agents speeding up metabolism and biochemical reactions. The same category includes also natural stimulants such as coffee, citrus fruit, green tea, nuts and the like. The agents can also be purely chemical constituents producing a great effect but being extremely dangerous to a body in return for a careless approach to them. These are such medications as thyroxine, dinitrophenol, xenical, etc.
2. The second option is split meals. It implies the principle of cheating a body. On the one hand, we speed up metabolism using this method. On the other hand, we eat small portions with a lack of total amount of calories.

ACTIVE ENERGY EXPENDITURE

Active expenditure is all you spend apart from the passive energy expenditure. That is, the actions which do not directly support the sustenance of a body are performed. Everything we do, including visiting the barber shop, repairing plumbing fixtures in the house or even typing, is an example of active expenditure. All the physical activity requiring energy fits the description of active expenditure. If a person tries to choose certain physical exercises to lose weight, he or she just fills the deficiency of active expenditure, not creates it. Recalling the example of muscular guys, we realize how much effort we need to acquire sufficient muscle mass, where the fat will not be deposited with your common food intake. At the same time, a low-calorie diet seems faster and more rational in terms of time and effort.

We speak not about failure or meaninglessness of exercises for weight loss, we speak rather about their smaller effectiveness comparing to the correct diet. If you increase the number of sets or a working weight in a gym, it will contribute less to fat burning. On the contrary, you will launch a growth effect in such a way. All you do with weights is primarily aimed at anabolism, not at weight loss which is catabolism. Thus, a person who wants to lose weight should be engaged in just losing weight for the moment. Meanwhile, a person who wants to gain muscle mass should be engaged exclusively in gaining it. It is impossible to become larger and smaller at the same time as it is absurd in nature.

When viewed in the context of physical activity, we distinguish between power load, exercises with weights, aerobics, endurance training with minimum load or your own weight. It is clear that we will spend fewer calories when doing exercises with weights if compared to the same time running on a treadmill. Here we have two principles of energy consumption. If we lift heavy weights, the carbohydrates are used as fuel. If we run, the fat cells are used as fuel. In this case, it is clear that it is better to run if you want to get rid of fat. If you want to increase muscles, weights will help you.

Now think of the following thing: both the first and the second option of loads, if done at a sufficient period of time, will take away 200 - 400 calories from you, which is absolutely not enough for normal stable weight loss. So, it is the diet which becomes a clear priority for the weight loss, not just increase in physical activity. Let's consider another misconception regarding spiking strength levels and fat burning.

This misconception concerns the exercises for selective targeting certain body parts. Constantly working out abs to the point of exhaustion will not help your body get rid of the excess fat in the abdominal area if your diet habits are wrong. Fat spreads throughout the body where it finds it convenient to and it does not ask a person where he or she wanted to store it. If the body processes are not fully tuned for burning fat, it is simply impossible to get rid of fat in certain body parts. Let's summarize:

- Lack of calories can provoke weight loss;
- Physical exercises themselves are ineffective without a diet, reducing the intake of calories.

Chapter 2. Types and Peculiarities of Diets

Let's first sort out the principles of correct dieting on the example of their wrong perception and use. We should do this in order to properly perceive the following list of the types of diets.

Mistake 1:

This mistake is rather popular among the girls trying to lose weight as quickly as possible. Very often you can hear about the diets which forbid everything except just one product. For example, a diet allowing intake of a single ingredient: apple, kiwi and so on. It will clearly cause a really big restriction on the number of calories per day, but what will be the result? Typically, these murderous diets lead the body to launch of reserve sources of energy beyond fat deposits. That is, the body will partially take energy from fat deposits, but it will also save energy by reducing the size of internals and slowing down cerebration. Such a diet will result in a flabby body, still having fat, and a terrible feeling, often painful and requiring rehabilitation.

Mistake 2:

People sometimes perceive diet as limiting "harmful" products, not calories. They just stop eating fried foods, processed food, fast food products and replacing them with boiled, useful dietetic foods such as buckwheat, rice, or potatoes without taking into account their weight when consumed. Some people think that eating healthy food is enough to burn fat. This is fundamentally wrong, because if you eat a lot of useful food, you can get the same amount of calories when eating a Big Mac. The main thing is to **CONTROL CALORIE INTAKE** while eating useful products.

Partially correct actions are not absolutely correct. When it comes to losing weight, you cannot gain the result by taking many partially correct steps or adhering to a partially effective plan. Everything should be clearly itemized and counted. You should observe strict proportionality of eaten products, be aware of their calorie content. Many people think that their feelings will help them understand the correct amount of food they eat to lose weight. DO NOT DELUDE YOURSELF! Your body will definitely deceive you. On the contrary, the exact calorie counting will not misguide you.

In such cases, people usually do not get the result or it is extremely low. After all, they cannot say exactly how many calories they got yesterday or today, hence, they cannot regulate the process. We should keep strict count from the zero point until the last day of being on a diet.

ZERO POINT (STARTING POINT)

You should mark a starting point at the beginning of the path heading to a fit body. You should understand where you start your way and what your destination is. It is clear that you can weigh yourself to understand what you should work with and when the weight will start to reduce. However, this will not help you understand what quantity of calories has caused the situation, forcing you to be on a chosen diet. There is a logical question - how to assess the starting point? We will not speculate on possible options but immediately offer the most effective way.

You should draw a primitive chart in a notebook or create it in an electronic file in order to accurately determine , in calories, which indicators you start from to achieve a certain goal. The chart includes just four parameters:

- date;
- personal weight;
- products you eat;
- caloric value of meals taken.

The first day of the diet you should weigh yourself in the morning and weigh and write down all the meals taken during the day. It's your task for five days. Day six, indicate the calorie content of all the products you ate the previous five days, including a number of proteins, fats, and carbohydrates, taking into account the weight of products. You can count the calories using the charts of calorie consumption which widely represented on the Internet. Each day is counted separately. Then, the amount of calories per each day is summed together and divided by five to determine the average number of calories consumed at the starting point.

MANAGING THE WEIGHT LOSS

Now that you have learned what quantity of calories is normal for you, you should make a list of products for the period of the whole diet to better control the process of losing weight. You should eat the same food products throughout the diet as this will help to maximize control over the situation and the process as a whole. Once the diet is chosen, let's start to lose weight and adjust the results.

After you have defined the starting point during the first week, the next day you should remove the part of calories in the form of a quantity of consumed products for the entire following week. Do not forget to continue to write down the personal weight, the meals taken and the calories consumed in your chart. The next week you should adjust the number of calories for a stable, safe weight loss, depending on your results. This should be done as follows:

- If you lose 1-2.65 pounds during a week, it's a good result so continue to stick to your chosen eating habits to achieve the result.
- If your weight loss is at a standstill, reduce calories taken even more.
- If you lose 6-11 pounds during the first week, you urgently need to increase food intake, otherwise you will provoke a slowdown of metabolism with subsequent "rollback" after the diet is over.

To make diet adjustments comfortable for your body while adding or removing some products, you should use complex carbohydrates: buckwheat, oatmeal, or rice, relying on your diet.

WHAT YOU SHOULD EAT DURING THE DIET

Undoubtedly, the best rule in the majority of diets is the complete elimination of fatty foods. Different food products have a greater or lesser benefit for weight loss. To make a fat burning process much more efficient, choose the right products. The products must be boiled, no fried foods, to retain all their beneficial properties and contain fewer calories. Apart from fat, you should reduce the intake of carbohydrates, which are abundantly represented in sweets, bread, and even vegetables. Therefore, if you aim at weight loss, it is necessary to mutually reduce the intake of fats and carbohydrates.

However, there is a peculiarity regarding the carbohydrates. Meanwhile, we definitely require no fats to lose weight, the carbohydrates will be useful enough. The question is what type of carbohydrates we mean. The quick-release carbohydrates (chocolate, sugar, honey, all possible sweet supplements) rapidly deposit in fat cells by increasing the level of insulin in the blood. The slow-release carbohydrates, generally contained in plant foods (fruit, vegetables, oatmeal, rice, etc.), do not cause a significant surge of insulin and contribute to the buildup of fat to a lesser extent. The latter products (fruit and vegetables) are also rich in fiber, which slows down the absorption of carbohydrates making the "energy" reserves. Thus, it is very important to use the slow-release carbohydrates in your diet giving priority to vegetables.

PROTEINS AS BUILDING BLOCKS OF A BODY

While removing fatty foods from your diet, reducing the quantity of food with quick-release carbohydrates, you should still keep the main building blocks of your body – the proteins. The high-molecular biological substances called proteins influence the construction of all tissues of a body, without exception. That is, being a major building block for a body, protein is extremely useful for maintaining and gaining muscle mass. In addition, the intake of protein does not cause a surge of insulin which makes us gain bad-quality weight. Therefore, it becomes obvious why many athletes increase the intake of chicken breasts, eggs and lean meat rich in protein. Eat a lot of protein during your diet!

CONCLUSION

Resting on the above-mentioned, you should get rid of fatty foods, replacing them with a large number of protein analogs, and consume slow-release carbohydrates in small quantities to get positive and correct results during your diet. As a moral support and diversity of taste, you can eat vegetables which will not adversely affect your results because of high fiber content.

DIET CHOICE

All kinds of diets effective for weight loss use a basic principle of limiting the calories taken in. The most efficient diets ban quick-release carbohydrates and fats to reduce stimulation of insulin secretion, and hence, accumulation of fat deposits. Yet there are exceptions to the rule, so we can highlight three main types of diets.

CYCLIC DIET

The trick of this diet is a dramatic change of daily intakes from low-calorie and carbohydrate-free diet to high-carbohydrate diet. A specific scheme of this diet is food intake with a minimum of calories and almost no carbohydrates during five days and saturating a body with carbohydrates during next two days. The principle of operation is as follows: body starts to lose weight at a critical shortage of carbohydrates, and two days of unrestrained absorption of carbohydrate are required to launch (speed up) metabolism. We know that if a body is starving for a long time, it shuts down and starts to give power very badly. To prevent this from happening, we deceive it with two days of oversupply, making it speed up metabolism.

A certain drawback of this diet is that it is more suitable for experienced bodybuilders. The fact is that everybody is unique and peculiarities of metabolism and perception of the diet may be different. Some people will find 5/2 mode suitable while 3/2 or 4/1mode will become a wonderful option for others. It depends on how quickly a body begins to reduce the energy output and what kind of response it has to a large number of carbohydrates. The concept of large or insufficient amounts of carbohydrates is different for each person. Someone eats a chocolate bar and starts to gain weight while someone needs a triple serving of fried fatty meat to get a slight change in weight. This adjustment is extremely difficult for beginners that do not yet feel the body's response to certain actions.

LOW-CARB DIET

This type of diet is clear but requires a stable output without any drops as in the previous option. You should remove completely all fats from your diet and begin to consume large amounts of animal protein from meat, fish, and eggs, as well as products with a minimum amount of slow-release carbohydrates. Afterward, having defined the eating habits which suit you most, you start to strictly adhere to them day by day, weighing yourself and determining the caloric value of meals eaten during the day. Depending on the effect happening to you during the week, adjust the process of losing weight in the way it was described previously. This type of diet can be considered quite suitable for the majority, but be responsible with regard to the calculations.

KETOGENIC DIET

We have often encountered in our practice a rather absurd question - how to lose weight eating fatty meat, kabobs and all foods we love so much? In fact, this question has an answer. There is a way to lose weight by eating high-fat foods and it is extremely effective. The body's usual sources of energy are carbohydrates, and it is enough for a body to work just having these substances. However, if you completely remove carbohydrate foods from your diet, your body will launch a process called ketosis.

Ketosis makes fat divide into acids and ketone bodies. A body uses the latter as the energy source. A body literally eats the fat cells. What could be better than eating the most delicious fatty foods and still lose weight? However, it is extremely difficult for your body to do as it is something the body is not accustomed to working with. Your state of health and work of digestive system will be quite unusual. The complete rebuilding of the internal sustenance system requires substantial loads on a body, so this should be taken into account when choosing this type of diet.

WHAT SHOULD BE CHOSEN?

As we have already mentioned when specifying the diets, you should analyze in details the diet you want to choose, either it would be a ketogenic or a cyclic diet. YOU SHOULD SERIOUSLY EVALUATE YOUR KNOWLEDGE! The low-carb diet will be definitely the best option for beginners or people with an average level of training. It is simple and accessible, not only in the perception of numbers and action sequences but is much easier for the body to perceive. People often make a common mistake when waiting for something for a long time, tolerating and then trying to achieve maximum results in a short time. This approach may give certain results, but choosing a well-balanced option is often the most proven and reliable way.

If drawing an analogy between speed and result, it is possible to give an example of elasticity and tone of muscles. When we lift weights in the gym, we feel the muscles swelling, becoming larger and relief at the end of the workout. But the muscles decline, taking their natural form immediately after we cool off. However, if we do work out in the gym for a long period of time, the maximum size of the muscles we have at the end of the workout will become natural in a calm state over some time. So, in terms of diet, we recommend a low-carb diet as a tool for sustainable and safe weight loss.

Chapter 3. Food for Result

We have come to the largest chapter, which gives precise pieces of advice on eating habits for men and women of different body types for stable and healthy weight loss. It should be noted that we have elaborated the plans in which the average consumption of calories is calculated for three categories of people. We are saying that in no instance will they suit everyone perfectly, as this is impossible. Each person is unique, and the number of calories required for the best effect will most likely differ. However, the main points of the diet adjustment have been revealed earlier, so the attentive readers will have no difficulties with calculations. Later on, it is important to remember how to determine and adjust the starting point when applying one of three plans.

Pay special attention to this chapter as it contains 70% of your success!

Three healthy meal plans for weight loss

When planning meal plans for different categories of people, we have attempted to provide information about the most common problem groups. The meals plans are divided into the work with such categories of people: men weighing 155-175 lb. with common energy expenditure; women with natural weight of 130 lb.; men weighing over 175 lb. with an increased need for energy. The numbers are taken on the basis of average data for each category and cannot be a reference since it would require an individual analysis of each individual reader.

Therefore, these indicators are more suitable for rapid selection of the meal plan priorities. Later, during the diet, we will adjust, increase or decrease your calorie intake according to the above-mentioned principles. The main information is of common nature for three plans, and it makes no sense to repeat these aspects. Therefore, the first option will provide the most detailed information, which is also important for the second and the third plans. In case the first plan does not suit you because of sex or weight, you still need to read it.

MEAL PLAN FOR MEN WEIGHING 155-176 POUNDS (WITH COMMON ENERGY EXPENDITURE OF 1,500-2,000 KCAL)

At the beginning of our way, let's select the right products for 2,000 kcal per day.

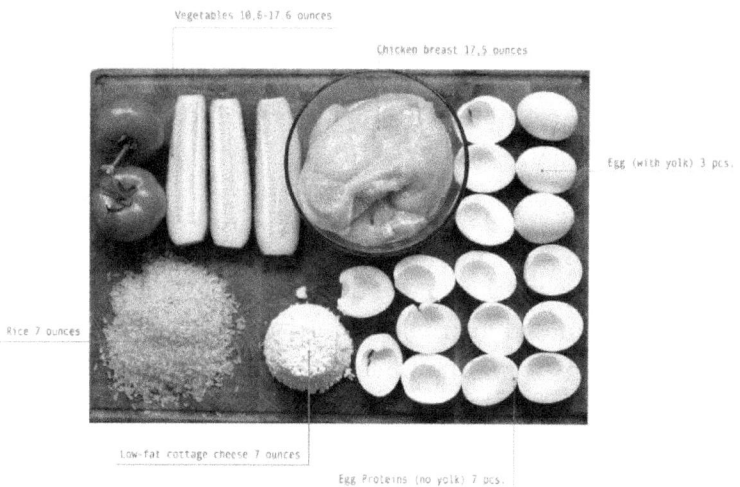

Products for the day:
- Chicken breast 17,5 oz = 3,5 oz of protein + 600 kcal
- Egg Proteins (no yolk) 7 pcs. = 1,4 oz protein + 154 kcal
- Rice 7 oz = 5,36 oz carbohydrates + 690 kcal
- Egg (with yolk) 3 pcs. = 0,95 oz protein + 330 kcal

- Vegetables 10,6-17,6 oz = 0,5-0,7 oz carbohydrates + 70-100 kcal
- Low-fat cottage cheese 7 oz = 1,3 oz protein + 192 kcal

Total: 6 oz of carbohydrate + 7 oz of protein equaling about 2,000 kcal

Extra information on foods:

- Everything is boiled
- Only chicken breasts are taken and no other parts
- Eggs are the largest that can be found
- Rice is weighed dry
- 0% fat cottage cheese
- If you need to reduce your calorie intake per day, do this at the expense of rice
- In case you are very hungry and are close to the edge, you can increase portions at the expense of egg whites

Divide the ingredients for the daily intake as follows:

- Rice is divided into four equal portions of 1,8 oz
- Chicken breast are divided into four equal portions of 5,3 oz
- Vegetables are divided into the number of intakes suitable for you

Foods peculiarities:

- Egg whites excellently compensate for food shortages. They can be eaten in large quantities with no negative consequences.

The better control over the process you have during the diet, the easier it will be to adjust its results. The correct approach to the food intake during the day is cooking in advance for the whole day in the morning or in the evening. You should prepare your meals for the whole coming day and proportionally divide the calories into food intakes. It will be much more useful for your body if you eat in small portions as often as possible during the day.

You should have a minimum of six meals in this kind of diet. This is done in order to create an illusion of a stable abundance of external energy supplies to your body. To put it simply, if your body eats often, it thinks that there are no problems in getting food and spends its fat deposits, which it thinks are easily replenished. On the contrary, if we decide to eat once or twice a day, the body realizes that it is difficult to obtain food for us and it should save its fat deposits, reducing energy expenditure. Therefore, you should divide the daily ration into plastic containers (first breakfast, second breakfast, lunch, afternoon snack, first dinner, second dinner). In addition, do not forget about the post-exercise carbohydrates and cottage cheese before going to bed which we do not consider to be food intakes.

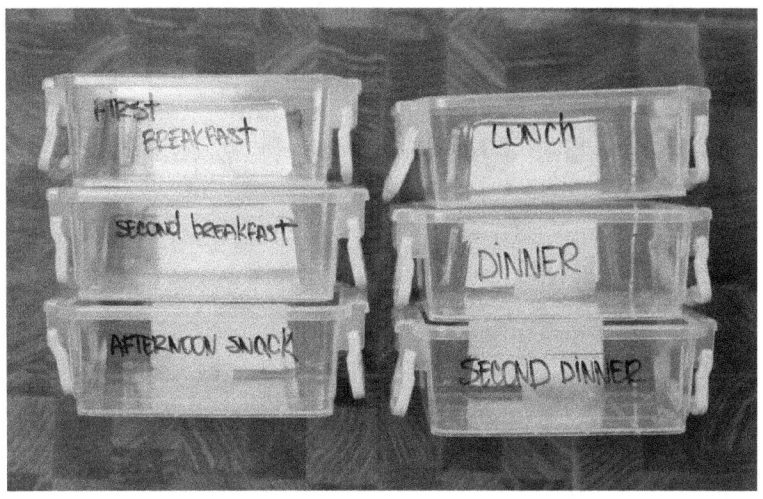

We have also prepared two alternative plans for people not fond of chicken breast, or those who would like a more varied menu:

Beef & Fish plan

- Rice 7 oz = + 5,3 oz carbohydrates + 690 kcal
- Lean beef 10,6 oz = 2,1 oz protein + 560 kcal
- Fish Cod 7 oz = 1,1 oz protein + 138 kcal
- Egg Proteins (no yolk) 7 pcs. = 1,4 oz protein + 154 kcal
- Egg (with yolk) 3 pcs. = 0,95 oz protein + 170 kcal
- Vegetables 10,6-17,6 oz = 15-20 carbohydrates + 70 - 100 kcal

Total: 6 oz of carbohydrate + 7,1 oz of protein equaling about 2,100 kcal

Note: Do not forget that beef is fattier than chicken and its choice should be given special attention.

Fish plan

- Rice 7 oz = 5,4 oz of carbohydrates + 690 kcal
- Fish Pollock 32 oz = 5,1 oz of protein + 621 kcal
- Egg (no yolk) 12 pcs. = 2,4 oz of protein + 264 kcal
- Low-fat cottage cheese 11 oz = 2 oz protein + 288 kcal
- Vegetables 10,6-17,6 oz = 15-20 carbohydrates + 70 - 100 kcal

Total: 6 oz of carbohydrate + 9,3 oz of protein equaling about 2,000 kcal

Food intake schedule:

8:00 a.m. – Morning

8:05 a.m. – Half glass of water or juice

8:20 a.m. – First breakfast: 1,8 oz of rice + 5,3 oz of chicken + vegetables

11:00 a.m. – Second breakfast: 1,8 oz of rice + 2 egg whites + one whole egg + vegetables

1:00 p.m. – Lunch: 1,8 oz of rice + 5,3 oz of chicken + vegetables

3:00 p.m. – Afternoon snack: two eggs without yolk + one whole egg + vegetables

5:00 p.m. - 06:00 p.m. – Workout

6:05 p.m. – Fast release protein, amino acids or one egg white + one whole egg

7:00 p.m. – Dinner: 1,8 oz of rice + 5,3 oz of chicken + vegetables

9:00 p.m. – Second dinner: 5,3 oz of chicken + two egg whites + vegetables

11:40 p.m. – 7 oz of cottage cheese before going to bed

11: 50 p.m. - 08:00 a.m. – Bedtime

Minute-by-minute day schedule

Here is a sample schedule based on the first, the standard meal plan. If you use an alternative plan, it won't be difficult to follow it using this algorithm.

8:00 a.m. – Getting up marks a new productive day and should be followed with a glass of pure cool water. Wash up and start to prepare the meals for the day ahead awakening the body completely.

8:20-8:30 a.m. – Your long-awaited first breakfast consists of 1,8 oz of rice, 5,3 oz of chicken breast and vegetables (tomatoes, cucumbers - to your liking). Prepare your meal containers before leaving for work, studies, and so on.

11:00 a.m. – Second breakfast consists of 1,8 oz of rice, two eggs without yolk + one whole egg and vegetables to your liking. Get used to eating in the most unexpected places – in the classrooms during the break, in a taxi, on a building site, etc.

1:00 p.m. – Lunch is a productive time to burn calories. You already feel a lack of energy having a big desire to eat, slight weakness is also possible. The shortage is partially compensated with 1,8 oz of rice, 5,3 oz of chicken breast and vegetables.

3:00 p.m. – Afternoon snack is the last food intake before a workout. This choice of food will have a particularly productive impact on your workout. For your body to consume fats and not to destroy muscles due to the shortage of energy during the intensive exercises, you should stock up with easy protein by eating two eggs without the yolks, one whole egg, and some vegetables. Thus, we get good amino acids without damaging the muscles with hungry exercise, but making it disintegrate the fat cells.

5:00 p.m. - 06:00 p.m. – Workout

6:05 p.m. – Take fast release protein literally immediately after the workout, not leaving the gym, so that your heated body would not consume the muscles because of lack of energy. Branched-chain amino acids or one egg without the yolk + one whole egg are the perfect options.

7:00 p.m. – First dinner. Carbohydrate replenishment is needed not to exacerbate the feeling of lack of calories. The first dinner repeats the breakfast: 1,8 oz of rice, 5,3 oz of chicken and vegetables to your liking. It will be the last intake of carbohydrates for today because later your body tends to sleep, and therefore thinks it no longer needs energy today and should put it off for tomorrow in the form of fat.

9:00 p.m. – Second dinner. Everything is simple. We cannot take carbohydrates, so we eat 5,3 oz of chicken, two eggs without the yolks and vegetables.

11:40 p.m. – Slow protein is the best meal option before going to bed to keep your basic expenditure at night. You may take casein-based protein. However, the more natural food is preferable, such as a serving of 7 oz of cottage cheese.

11: 50 p.m. - 08:00 a.m. – Sleep

Tips:

Of course, the most common right advice of all fitness trainers is to drink as much water as possible. We will not delve into the details of percentage ratio of the water composition in the human body, just once again confirm that the water is an integral part of the process of the weight loss and life in general. The trainees also ask often what they should do if the workout takes place not at the time specified in the schedule. Everything is simple, we need only to follow the plan: take more carbohydrates in the morning, more proteins in the evening, and take fast release protein after the workout.

It may surprise you, but people obtained the opportunity to assimilate dairy products just a couple of thousand years ago in the course of their evolution. Primarily, the genome unit responsible for such an assimilation appeared in the steppe peoples who were forced to adapt to new conditions due to the lack of nutrients. Nowadays, many adults often poorly digest lactose, so if you feel during the diet that you do not assimilate cottage cheese, you can easily replace it with the night protein or ten egg whites.

MEAL PLAN FOR WOMEN (WITH COMMON ENERGY EXPENDITURE OF 1,000-1,500 KCAL)

The day and meal schedule for girls and women actually does not differ from the men's schedule, except for the lower level of calories in the diet. The selection of products, adjustment of the calories during the week, noting down the weight and the selected products – everything should be done in the same sequence and with the same thoroughness. The female body has its own peculiarities as one of the main natural tasks of women is childbirth, so the female body is programmed to accumulate fats for an emergency. Like any other human feature, this is reasoned by the evolution and is a response to the life of our ancestors living hundreds and thousands of years ago.

Another consequence of the evolutionary process is that a woman has smaller muscle mass, which, as we remember, allows losing weight easily. It is another spoke in the wheel of fast weight loss for women. The physiological characteristics of muscles make it clear that if a man weighs 200 lb, a ratio of his muscle mass to his weight is significantly bigger than that of a woman with the same weight. We understand that she has excess fat, which she should ruthlessly get rid of. However, do not forget about the harmful effects of especially intensive calorie reduction as it is not only harmful to health but also slows down the fat burning process.

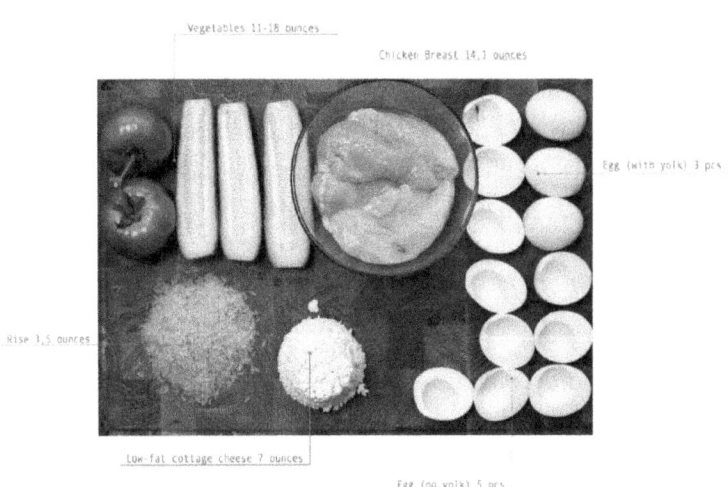

Meal plan for women:
- Rise 3,5 oz. = 2,7 oz. of carbohydrates + 345 kcal
- Chicken Breast 14,1 oz. = 2,8 oz. of protein + 480 kcal
- Egg (no yolk) 5 pcs. = 1 oz. of protein + 110 kcal
- Egg (with yolk) 3 pcs. = 1,3 oz. of protein + 330 kcal

- Low-fat cottage cheese 7 oz. = 1,3 oz. protein + 192 kcal
- Vegetables 10,6-17,6 oz. = 15-20 carbohydrates + 70-100 kcal

Total: 3,5 oz. of carbohydrate + 6 oz. of protein equaling about 1,500 kcal

Tips:

Knowing the overall women's love for all kinds of sweets, we should clarify and remind you that if you want to achieve results, it is necessary to adhere to strict compliance with the list of products included in your diet. You cannot supplement your daily diet with biscuits, yogurt, sweets, etc. Still, the diet can be varied with the products you will find immediately after the last meal plan. We want to protect particularly zealous ladies from the desire to lose weight within the shortest possible period of time. Both the male and female body has a negative reaction to losing weight due to a sharp decrease in calories.

The weight loss of 17,6 oz. will be a normal week result for the women. If it is 2,2 lb., it is a perfect result. However, if a woman loses over 2,2 lb., she should increase the calorie intake per day immediately. You should also take into account the impact of periods causing changes in weight. A jump in weight may occur few days before the period but the weight will return to normal after they end. A woman should be ready for that and should not blame incorrect drawing up of a meal plan.

MEAL PLAN FOR MEN WEIGHING OVER 180 LB. (WITH CONSIDERABLE ENERGY EXPENDITURE OF 2,000-2,500 KCAL)

There is no sense to hold forth on the points we have described in the first plan as they differ only in portions. This plan is for people requiring high daily energy consumption, for example, people working in long shifts at the factory, miners, programmers writing the complex algorithms for 16 hours, or simply people with big muscle mass.

Meal plan for men weighing over 180 lb.
- Rise 10,6 oz. = 8 oz. of carbohydrates + 1030 kcal
- Chicken Breast 21 oz. = 4,2 oz. of protein + 720 kcal
- Egg (no yolk) 7 pcs. = 1,4 oz. of protein + 154 kcal
- Egg (with yolk) 3 pcs. = 1 oz. of protein + 330 kcal
- Low-fat cottage cheese 7 oz. = 1,3 oz. of protein + 192 kcal
- Vegetables 10,6-17,6 oz. = 15-20 carbohydrates + 70-100 kcal

Total: 8,8 oz. of carbohydrate + 7,9 oz. of protein equaling about 2,500 kcal

Tips:
If your weight significantly exceeds 180 lb., you are likely to feel slight hunger during the first days of your diet. It still happens that people even with such a weight feel full at the end of the day instead of slight starvation. In some cases, it is still better to apply a general plan for the men weighing up to 180 lb. to adjust the necessary supply of calories to the body as quickly as possible.

Foods for variety:
- Protein (in 3,5 oz. of food)
- Chicken Breast = 0,7 oz. of protein + 120 kcal
- Egg (with yolk) 1pcs. = 0,3 oz. of protein + 0,2 oz. of fat + 88 kcal

- Egg (no yolk) 5 pcs. = 1 oz. of protein + 110 kcal
- Beef = 0,7 oz. of protein + 0,4 oz. of fat + 187 kcal
- Beef heart = 0,5 oz. of protein + 87 kcal
- Cod or pollack = 0,6 oz. of protein + 69 kcal
- Milk 1% = 0,1 oz. of protein + 37 kcal
- Low-fat cottage cheese = 0,6 oz. of protein + 96 kcal
- Night protein = 2,1-2,8 oz. of protein + 350 kcal

Carbohydrates (in 3,5 oz. of food)

- Potatoes = 0,7 oz. of carbohydrates + 87 kcal
- Rice = 2,7 oz. of carbohydrates + 345 kcal
- Oat groats = 2,4 oz. of carbohydrates + 345 kcal
- Buckwheat = 2,4 oz. of carbohydrates + 345 kcal
- Grapefruit = 0,2 oz. of carbohydrates + 32 kcal
- Grapes = 0,6 oz. of carbohydrates +85 kcal
- Orange = 0,3 oz. of carbohydrates + 37 kcal
- Bananas = 0,8 oz. of carbohydrates = 94 kcal

SAFE BOOSTERS FOR FAT LOSS

If you crave additional stimulation for the body to speed up fat burning, you may use additives allowing to achieve your tasks quickly. We will not create an encyclopedia, just offer you the most popular, safe and affordable ones.

Levocarnitine

This additive has two positive effects during your dieting. The first is an improvement of digestion by increasing the secretion of the corresponding enzymes. Second, levocarnitine facilitates movement of the fat cells to the mitochondria which convert them into the energy. The duo of these effects excellently stimulates the body's energy metabolism and helps lose the excess body fat faster.

Guarana

This energy additive, which stimulates the noradrenaline secretion, creates an illusion of the energy surplus even in its absence. Stimulation occurs through the nervous system, making fat burn actively. The product's concentration of caffeine is higher than that of the coffee beans. The dangers and benefits of guarana equal those of the extremely strong coffee, so it is safe if it is not abused.

Omega-3

It is a great additive to the fat burning diet which is literally required by our body but which is produced only outside of it. It has a number of positive effects on the body such as stabilization of metabolic processes, improvement of the cardiovascular system, reduction in the inflammation prospects, protection of muscles against destruction. The main source of Omega-3 is fish and seafood, but nuts, legumes, spinach and leeks also contain it.

CHAPTER 4. MOVEMENT IS LIFE

Physical activity is the process of interaction of a body with the outside world by means of the reaction of the muscle fibers. This type of activity has a direct impact on building up of the muscle mass and regulation of the fat deposits in a body. Nowadays, there is a huge amount of very different types of physical activity, which help not only significantly increase the joint mobility, but to reduce the risk of various musculoskeletal system diseases as well.

Speaking more generally, the physical activity can be divided into several types:

- Aerobic activity or cardio workout has a positive effect on the muscle group and on the cardiovascular system. The basic exercises include jogging, exercycle, skipping rope, etc.;
- Anaerobic activity (workout with weights).

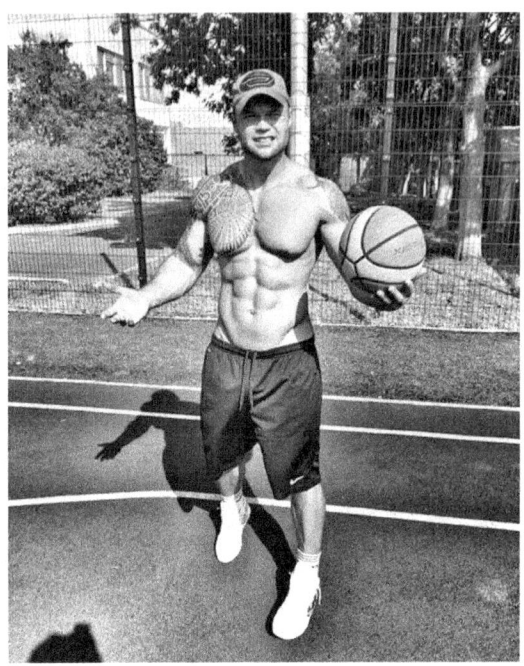

Many people wonder what activity they should choose to achieve the best possible results. The answer is very simple: you need to combine exercises! This aspect will help you to achieve the incredible results within the shortest possible time. The fact is that each load has its specific features necessary for weight loss. Let's study the most energy-consuming kind of load – CARDIO exercises, which make the fat burn.

You do the exercises producing the load on the cardiovascular system at the end of your workout when you will have already spent a huge amount of CARBOHYDRATES that has been received during the day (few days). So do not goof off in the gym as unspent carbohydrates (energy) will remain in the body stocks and then turn into fat tissue, which you and I are fighting so hard against. It should also be noted that the anaerobic activity creates a greater calorie deficit compared to the aerobic activity because the muscles need not only time but also extra energy in order to restore the damaged muscle fibers.

POWER LOAD (WORKOUT WITH WEIGHTS)

Power load is the integral part of any training as the exercises with the gym weights build up an attractive and sexy body. How should you work out for shredding? Typically, most people include a huge number of sets, repetitions, and supersets in their program in order to achieve this goal. Of course, this makes sense, you only need to know how to put it to work as the unreasonable use of such techniques can hurt your body.

The fact is that the load power causes consumption of the large amounts of carbohydrates and a body naturally begins to look for the energy in order to replenish the stocks thus combusting the muscle tissue. To avoid such unpleasant moments, take branched-chain amino acids, which will provide your muscles with additional energy. If you are not a supporter of sports nutrition, you need to analyze your body a bit. If you see that your muscles develop normally after weight training, do not load them, even more, to "squeeze out" a maximum. Adhere to your usual program and put more emphasis on CARDIO exercises to burn fat to obtain the perfect body.

TIPS ABOUT AEROBIC ACTIVITY

If you want to try harder, this type of activity is exactly what you need! It is a perfect way to burn fat and strengthen the cardiovascular system. The essence is very simple: you need to perform repetitive movements (running, exercycle, skipping rope, brisk walking, etc.) of low intensity. Why do you need exactly low intensity? If we train with a light load, it is more convenient for our body to produce energy in "cheap" ways through the oxidation of fat. If you start to increase the pace of cardio, this chemical process will be changed by a body and a body will start to burn carbohydrates instead of fat tissue. It is, therefore, necessary to keep the low pace for a rather long period of time (up to one hour).

To further accelerate the process, you need to follow such guidelines: you should do a cardio workout when your body contains a minimal amount of carbohydrates as this will make your body switch to fat burning.

What is the best time for CARDIO exercises? There are several favorable periods:

- in the morning (immediately after awakening when your body has no carbohydrates because you have not eaten);
- after workout (carbohydrate stocks are spent during the power load);
- before bedtime (lack of carbohydrates caused by protein intake).

Which option is the best? Each has its pros and cons. If you want to burn as much fat as possible, the ideal option would be the cardio workout in the morning and the weight training in the day time. This method is "murderous" for the fat tissue. As for the advantages of CARDIO exercises before the bedtime, your body will create a "fat burning background" which will be very useful if you do not indulge in carbohydrates in the evening. The advantage of CARDIO exercises after the main workout is convenience, since it is not necessary to carry out the second training session breaking your day.

However, we should note specific cases when the common walking will be a good option for losing weight. This refers to people suffering from a particularly large number of "energy stocks" or people who have bad health. People weighing over 275 lb. are in a major hazard group with poor cardiac performance. Therefore, it is simply dangerous to listen to the pseudo trainers who make such people run around the stadium. Moreover, unusual physical activity destroys the joints and will, not to mention that the effect will not be commensurate with the effort.

Speaking of the overwork, just imagine throwing an extra load of 90 lb. (whether it will be weights, bags or fat) on an athlete with a normal muscle weight of 200 lb. Will it be easy? Therefore, untrained people may just walk. The main thing is that you personally feel these efforts and they will really lead you to the desired numbers on the scales. But do not forget that your body is getting used to the load and it should be increased. Even if you start to walk, increase walking pace gradually, finally progressing to jogging. Do not forget about the carbohydrate burning effect, which we do not seek.

REMEMBER: SLOW AND MEDIUM PACE BURNS FAT, FAST PACE BURNS CARBOHYDRATES.

RECOMMENDATIONS FOR THE SCHEME "CARDIO EXERCISES ON THE EMPTY STOMACH IN THE MORNING"

This method is very fitting when you need to lose weight quickly. However, you need to be very careful as the muscles may also start to burn in "hungry" conditions. To achieve the desired goal, you need to follow several very useful rules:

- do not eat (because carbohydrates "will block" fat burning process and you will have to spend   much more time on workout than usual);
- take pre-workout supplements (which speed up the energy expenditure during the exercises. If   you do not have this sports complex, you can then take a double coffee without sugar);
- keep low pace of workout (the goal is not speed, but duration to launch the oxidative processes   in the body);
- do not eat immediately after the cardio exercises as the longer you do not eat carbohydrates, the   longer your fat will burn. So, go to the shower slowly and then drink nutritional amino acids.

Listen constantly to your body during the workout. If you feel that your muscles start to "burn", you need to add little carbohydrates to your diet to help eliminate this negative process and achieve high results in fat loss.

CHAPTER 5. MINIMUM FAT, MAXIMUM MEAT

CONCLUSION

So, it's time to summarize. We hope that we have managed to convey the main aspects and principles of losing weight as well as to describe in detail the dieting and the accompanying changes in a body. Our experience shows that the most effective tool for getting a perfect body is primary, a die-hard desire to achieve your goal. In addition, this requires strict adherence to the chosen strategy without making any concessions to yourself and attempts to look for easier ways.

The endless advertisements of magic pills, miracle ointments and fitness equipment which do everything instead of you are the attempt of certain individuals to cash in on the positive aspirations of naive people. The result always requires your effort and patience. Even if you decide to take allegedly effective medicines, do not forget that rapid weight loss, which they may cause, will also require a kind of payback. So many inexperienced bodybuilders payback could not only be with the INCREASE in the old indicators of fat mass after taking the medicines but also with health as a token money in this case.

It is always up to you to decide, but first, think what you are ready to pay with for a slim body. Will it be the decrease in the normal activity of your body and an overall weakening of the immune system, or will it be the days and weeks of scrupulous low-carb dieting? Keep in mind that the healthy body is a top priority in losing weight. The ideal proportions are secondary though the much-desired product of this effort.

KEY TIPS

Follow properly the action sequence from the beginning to the end. Do not start to play with calories without defining your starting point, the common caloric intake prior to the diet. Do not make huge jerks after your caloric intake is reduced not to launch the defense mechanism of the body. Do not forget that the body is a zealous defender of its stocks and does not tolerate bullying. Eat boiled food, without diluting your diet with inappropriate candies, hot dogs and small portions of fried potatoes. Every piece of junk food, which you give up at the beginning of your diet, will become a huge stone to slow down your progress rate if you succumb.

A variety of food does not minimize the effect of diet, but only if you strictly adhere to the list of allowed products. Try to drink the maximum amount of water to improve the work of all the body systems. Drink water as often as possible, including 30 minutes before food intake. But remember it is desirable to drink water only 30 minutes **after** food intake. In doing so, we do not dilute the gastric juice with water, allowing it to carry out its work effectively. Do not forget about the importance of sleep in the process of metabolism. Monitor your results through weekly adjustment of the calorific value of the foods. Do not be lazy, keep a record of your progress and eaten foods, taking down the caloric value and the amount of carbohydrates and proteins.

PARTING WORDS

My colleague and I hope that this book will help many people to solve the issue of great importance for them. During our trainer career, we have succeeded in reshaping not only many dozens of human bodies, but many dozens of human minds as well, which is more important. The human power is not in muscles, it originates in what we call consciousness. The main goal of any exercise for a body is the ability of the consciousness to overcome your own imaginary obstacles and barriers imposed by the society.

Our main purpose is to show you in an accessible way that you are able to change, change for the better, in the direction you have chosen. All the obstacles are of conditional moral nature. There are many examples which we have seen with our eyes, that have inspired us and millions of people around, explaining that nothing is impossible. You just must say to yourself that there is nothing impossible for you. A human being gets a life not to live it as a spineless amoeba. We must marvel at life. We must see opportunities rather than obstacles and future results rather than current personal shortcomings.

All those people you admire and think they have reached incredible heights are the same people as you. There is no need to talk about the differences between there and your starting conditions. Believe me, a lot of those people who have become the best in their areas, professionals in sports or business, had far more modest possibilities than those you have now. Stop blaming bad weather, unstable economic situation, magnetic storms, your neighbor or anyone else, just pull yourself up and do what you need.

If you have picked up this book and read it from cover to cover, you have already started your path to victory. You have taken the first step on the way to the changes more serious than just a beautiful torso. You have risen to a higher level. You have become one point stronger and will become even stronger after you have complied with all the tips of this book. Close the door to the world of doubt, the world of deceit and self-pity. Fist your fear and uncertainty. The first thing you should do is to say loudly to yourself – Become a better person!

Good luck, friends!

About The Author

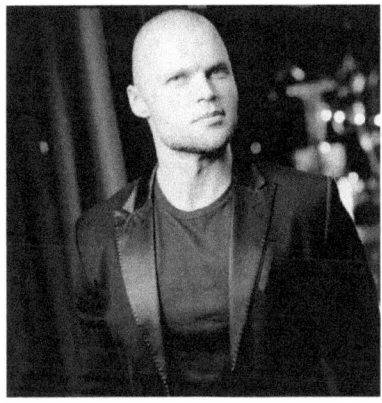

Edward Cruz is the #1 Amazon best-selling author of *How to lose belly fat: meal plans for ultimate weight loss for men and women in 8 weeks* among others. He lives in Chacago, Illinois with his family.

"I am not going to mislead you and promise that you will lose weight in a week - like many "teachers" do, while they cannot bring their own bodies in shape!

I will simply show you a working method that has helped me and many of my clients to keep our bodies toned and shaped at all times and achieve this in a fairly short time.

But the most important thing is that this technique will help you to lose weight at last and change your life forever!"

ONE LAST THING...

If you enjoyed this book or found it useful I'd be very grateful if you'd post a short review on Amazon. Your support really does make a difference and I read all the reviews personally so I can get your feedback and make this book even better.

If you'd like to leave a review then all you need to do is click the review link on this book's page on Amazon here:

I strongly believe that the advice in here can help people with their weight loss goals and you can help too by spreading the word.

If you think this book could be better in any way you can let me know what needs to be improved by sending an email to perfectecruz@gmail.com.

I can then update this and future books and provide he best information so that you and others can get even more value from this book.

Thanks again for your support!

www.ingramcontent.com/pod-product-compliance
Lightning Source LLC
Chambersburg PA
CBHW060649290526
45793CB00001B/470